Quantum Slimming

50 Revolutionary Superfoods that Defy Gravity and Melt Pounds away.

Tasha Mantr

Preface

Welcome to the book "Quantum Slimming," which ventures beyond the traditional approach to weight loss to explore the interplay between quantum physics and nutrition.

This groundbreaking book examines the power of 50 superfoods to impact weight loss and overall well-being.

Highlights of the book: 50 Superfoods:

- 50 Superfoods: Meticulously chosen superfoods are presented, each with its own unique properties and potential benefits for health and weight management.
- Science and Nutrition: The book delves into the science behind these superfoods, exploring their nutritional profiles and how they may interact with the body's systems.
- Real-Life Stories: Individuals who have incorporated these superfoods into their lifestyles share their personal experiences and outcomes.
- Holistic Approach: The book emphasizes the importance of a comprehensive approach to wellness, incorporating nutrition, lifestyle, and mindset.

Invitation to explore:

This book invites you to embark on a journey of discovery, exploring the power of these superfoods in terms of quantum consciousness. It is a guide to understanding the science behind these foods and the role they can play in leading a healthier and more vibrant lifestyle.

Join the search: Whether you're looking for a new way to lose weight or you're just curious about how quantum physics and nutrition fit together, this book offers a unique perspective and invites you to dive into the possibilities of research.

Discover your own path to wellness.

Let this book be the catalyst on your journey to a healthy, fulfilling life.

Table of Contents

Introduction

Within this book lies an extraordinary exploration into the remarkable fusion of quantum physics and nutrition.

Welcome to the world of "Quantum Slimming: 50 Revolutionary Superfoods That Defy Gravity and Melt Pounds Away." This groundbreaking book challenges the conventional ideologies surrounding weight loss by melding the principles of quantum mechanics with the transformative power of carefully selected superfoods.

Prepare yourself for a truly unique voyage towards wellness. As we delve into the intricacies of quantum physics and delve into the diverse qualities of 50 superfoods, the aim of this book is to present you with a fresh perspective on achieving a healthier lifestyle. The metaphorical theme of defying gravity pervades the narrative, symbolizing our departure from mundane weight loss approaches.

In the chapters that lie ahead, each superfood is not merely viewed as an ingredient but rather as a catalyst for change—a quantum leap in the quest for a healthier self. This culinary odyssey encourages you to reevaluate the limits of traditional diets and invites you to embark on a journey where science and nutrition beautifully intersect.

"Quantum Slimming" is an expedition into unexplored territory, challenging the ordinary to reinvent their approach to weight loss, regardless of how experienced they are in health and wellbeing.

So, buckle up, because we're about to undergo a quantum revolution. We accept a change that goes beyond the physical while on this journey, in addition to losing weight. Welcome to the quantum revolution of dieting, where the extraordinary becomes the new norm.

Chapter one
Unveiling Quantum Slimming

Greetings and welcome to the start of our Quantum Slimming adventure. In this chapter, we will explore quantum slimming, a novel and cutting-edge method of weight loss. Discard any physics preconceptions you may have; quantum slimming has nothing to do with formulas or cosmic forces. It involves reinventing how we view and accomplish weight loss by connecting it with the quantum nature of change.

1.1 Imagining a New Approach

Consider a weight loss approach that transcends the ordinary, a method not bound by conventional norms. Quantum slimming precisely introduces that—a departure from traditional weight loss strategies. This chapter invites you to imagine a world where the rules of the game are rewritten, opening new possibilities for achieving a healthier and more vibrant lifestyle.

1.2 A Fusion of Modern Concepts

So, what does quantum mean in quantum slimming? It's a metaphorical bridge between cutting-edge concepts and tangible results. The marriage of quantum ideas with weight loss principles is about embracing a modern and dynamic perspective. This section aims to demystify the notion of quantum in the context of slimming, making it accessible and applicable to our everyday lives.

1.3 Beyond Gravitational Metaphors

The phrase "Defying Gravity" isn't a literal escape from the earth's pull. Instead, it serves as a metaphor for transcending the gravitational forces that often hold us back in our weight-loss journeys. Quantum slimming challenges the gravitational pull of traditional methods, encouraging a shift in mindset towards a more effective and sustainable path to wellness.

1.4 Embracing a New Wellness Paradigm

Let go of any preconceived notions about quantum physics. Quantum slimming is a departure from the theoretical and a leap into a practical and applicable wellness paradigm.

This section unfolds the foundational concepts that guide us in this unconventional approach, setting the stage for a transformative journey.

1.5 The Quantum Slimming Promise

As we conclude this chapter, consider the promise of quantum slimming. It's not just another weight-loss method; it's a promise of embracing a holistic and achievable path to a healthier you. Quantum slimming holds the potential to redefine your relationship with weight loss, offering a fresh perspective and a practical guide for your wellness journey.

Stay tuned for Chapter 2, where we delve into the heart of quantum slimming—the 50 superfoods that will redefine how we nourish our bodies and defy the gravitational pull of excess weight.

Here is to embrace a new dimension in wellness!

Chapter Two
The Quantum Slimming Superfoods

In our exploration of "Quantum Slimming," this chapter brings us face-to-face with the heart of this transformative journey – the Quantum Slimming Superfoods. As a nutrition expert my goal is to shed light on the intricacies of each superfood, unraveling the unique nutritional profiles that contribute to their extraordinary role in defying gravity and aiding in weight loss.

2.1 Understanding the Quantum Slimming Selection Criteria

Before delving into the specifics of each superfood, it is essential to grasp the meticulous criteria employed in curating this list.

Quantum Slimming Superfoods are not arbitrary choices; rather, they are nutritional powerhouses meticulously selected for their extraordinary properties in defying gravity and aiding in weight loss. So, let's explore each of these 50 superfoods, understanding their unique contributions to our quantum quest.

2.2 The Quantum Slimming Superfoods Unveiled

Now, let us turn our attention to the stars of the show – the 50 superfoods that form the backbone of Quantum Slimming. Each one underwent a stringent selection based on its nutritional density, bioavailability, and proven weight loss benefits. This is not just an assembly of list, they are curated collections with intention and purpose… weight loss.

2.2.1 Avocado

Nutritional Profile:

Avocado is a nutrient-dense superfood rich in monounsaturated fats, which are heart-healthy fats. It also contains essential vitamins such as potassium, vitamin K, vitamin E, and B-vitamins.

Slimming Potential:

Satiety Boost: The healthy fats in avocados contribute to a feeling of fullness, helping control appetite and reduce overeating.

Metabolism Support: Monounsaturated fats may play a role in supporting a healthy metabolism.

Portion/Preparation:

 Aim for about half an avocado per serving. Incorporate it into salads, spreads, or enjoy it on its own for a satisfying snack.

2.2.2 Blueberries

Nutritional Profile:

Blueberries are packed with antioxidants, particularly anthocyanins, as well as vitamins C and K, and fiber.

Slimming Potential:

Antioxidant Power: The antioxidants in blueberries may help combat oxidative stress, potentially reducing inflammation and supporting overall health.

Fiber Boost: High fiber content contributes to satiety, aiding in appetite control.

Portion/Preparation:

A serving is typically one cup. Enjoy blueberries as a snack, in smoothies, or as a topping for yogurt or oatmeal.

2.2.3 Spinach

Nutritional Profile:

Spinach is a nutrient powerhouse, containing vitamins A, C, K, iron, calcium, and fiber.

Slimming Potential:

Low-Calorie Density: Spinach is low in calories but high in nutrients, making it an excellent choice for those looking to manage their weight.

Fiber Content: The fiber promotes a feeling of fullness and aids in digestion.

Portion/Preparation:

Include a generous handful in salads, smoothies, omelets, or as a side dish. Aim for at least one to two cups per serving.

2.2.4 Quinoa

Nutritional Profile:

Quinoa is a complete protein, containing all essential amino acids. It's also rich in fiber, magnesium, and various vitamins.

Slimming Potential:

Protein Prowess: The complete protein content supports muscle maintenance and may contribute to a feeling of fullness.

Complex Carbohydrates: The complex carbs in quinoa provide sustained energy, reducing the likelihood of energy crashes that can lead to overeating.

Portion/Preparation:

One cup of cooked quinoa is a standard serving. Use it as a base for salads, stir-fries, or as a side dish.

2.2.5 Kale

Nutritional Profile:

Kale is a nutrient-dense leafy green, high in vitamins A, C, and K, as well as calcium and fiber.

Slimming Potential:

Low-Calorie, High-Nutrient: Kale provides a wealth of nutrients with minimal calories, supporting weight management.

Fiber Content: Like spinach, the fiber in kale promotes a feeling of fullness and aids in digestion.

Portion/Preparation:

A serving is typically one to two cups. Enjoy kale in salads, smoothies, sautéed dishes, or as kale chips for a crunchy snack.

2.2.6 Chia Seeds

Nutritional Profile:

Chia seeds are rich in omega-3 fatty acids, fiber, protein, and various essential nutrients.

Slimming Potential:

Fiber Magic: Chia seeds expand when soaked, creating a gel-like consistency that promotes a feeling of fullness and aids digestion.

Protein Boost: The protein content supports muscle maintenance and can contribute to satiety.

Portion/Preparation:

A standard serving is around 1-2 tablespoons. Mix chia seeds into yogurt, oatmeal, or use them in smoothies. You can also make chia seed pudding by combining them with your choice of liquid.

2.2.7 Salmon

Nutritional Profile:

Salmon is fatty fish rich in omega-3 fatty acids, high-quality protein, vitamin D, and B-vitamins.

Slimming Potential:

Omega-3 Benefits: Omega-3s in salmon may help regulate appetite, reduce inflammation, and support metabolic health.

Protein Prowess: The high-quality protein supports muscle maintenance and contributes to a feeling of fullness.

Portion/Preparation:

A serving is typically around 3-4 ounces. Grill, bake, or poach salmon for a delicious and slimming main dish. Aim to include fatty fish like salmon in your diet at least twice a week.

2.2.8 Broccoli

Nutritional Profile:

Broccoli is a cruciferous vegetable rich in fiber, vitamins C and K, and various antioxidants.

Slimming Potential:

Fiber for Satiety: The fiber content promotes a feeling of fullness, aiding in portion control.

Nutrient Density: Broccoli is low in calories but high in nutrients, making it an excellent choice for weight management.

Portion/Preparation:

A serving is typically around one cup. Enjoy broccoli steamed, roasted, or as part of stir-fries and salads.

2.2.9 Almonds

Nutritional Profile:

Almonds are a nutrient-dense nut, providing healthy fats, protein, fiber, vitamin E, and magnesium.

Slimming Potential:

Satiety Powerhouse: The combination of healthy fats, protein, and fiber in almonds promotes a feeling of fullness.

Metabolism Support: Nutrients like magnesium may play a role in supporting a healthy metabolism.

Portion/Preparation:

A standard serving is around a small handful (about 1 ounce). Enjoy almonds as a snack, sprinkle them on salads, or incorporate them into your morning oatmeal or yogurt.

2.2.10 Sweet Potatoes

Nutritional Profile:

Sweet potatoes are rich in complex carbohydrates, fiber, vitamins A and C, and various minerals.

Slimming Potential:

Sustained Energy: The complex carbs provide sustained energy, reducing the likelihood of energy crashes and overeating.

Fiber Content: The fiber in sweet potatoes contribute to a feeling of fullness and supports digestive health.

Portion/Preparation:

A serving is typically one medium-sized sweet potato. Enjoy them baked, mashed, or roasted for a nutritious and satisfying side dish.

2.2.11 Cauliflower

Nutritional Profile:

Cauliflower is a cruciferous vegetable rich in fiber, vitamins C and K, and a variety of antioxidants.

Slimming Potential:

Low-Calorie Substitute: Cauliflower is a versatile, low-calorie alternative to starchy foods, making it ideal for those looking to manage their weight.

Fiber Boost: The fiber content supports digestive health and promotes a feeling of fullness.

Portion/Preparation:

A serving is typically around one cup. Enjoy cauliflower as a rice substitute, mashed as a potato alternative, or roasted for a flavorful side dish.

2.2.12 Greek Yogurt

Nutritional Profile:

Greek yogurt is a rich source of protein, probiotics, calcium, and essential vitamins.

Slimming Potential:

Protein Power: The high protein content in Greek yogurt supports muscle maintenance and contributes to a feeling of fullness.

Probiotic Benefits: Probiotics may promote gut health, potentially impacting weight regulation.

Portion/Preparation: A standard serving is around one cup. Enjoy Greek yogurt as a snack, in smoothies, or as a base for healthy parfaits.

2.2.13 Walnuts

Nutritional Profile:

Walnuts are a nutrient-dense nut, providing healthy fats, protein, fiber, and various vitamins and minerals.

Slimming Potential:

Heart-Healthy Fats: The omega-3 fatty acids in walnuts may support heart health and contribute to a feeling of fullness.

Satiety Booster: The combination of healthy fats and protein promotes satiety.

Portion/Preparation:

A standard serving is around a small handful (about 1 ounce). Enjoy walnuts as a snack, in salads, or add them to your morning oatmeal.

2.2.14 Oats

Nutritional Profile:

Oats are a whole grain rich in fiber, complex carbohydrates, and various vitamins and minerals.

Slimming Potential:

Satiety Support: The fiber and complex carbs in oats promote a feeling of fullness, aiding in appetite control.

Steady Energy: Oats provide sustained energy, reducing the likelihood of energy crashes and overeating.

Portion/Preparation:

A standard serving is around half to one cup. Enjoy oats as a hearty breakfast option, in smoothies, or as a base for healthy energy bars.

2.2.15 Beets

Nutritional Profile:

Beets are a root vegetable rich in antioxidants, fiber, vitamins, and minerals.

Slimming Potential:

Antioxidant Power: The antioxidants in beets may contribute to reducing inflammation, supporting overall health.

Fiber Content: Fiber supports digestive health and helps maintain a feeling of fullness.

Portion/Preparation:

A serving is typically around one cup. Enjoy beets roasted, boiled, or grated into salads for a nutritious and colorful addition.

2.2.16 Cacao

Nutritional Profile: C

acao is the raw form of chocolate, rich in antioxidants, flavonoids, and minerals like magnesium.

Slimming Potential:

Antioxidant Rich: The antioxidants in cacao may contribute to reducing oxidative stress, supporting overall health.

Mood and Energy Boost: Cacao contains compounds that may positively impact mood and provide a natural energy boost.

Portion/Preparation:

Incorporate cacao into smoothies, desserts, or enjoy it in its purest form by adding cacao nibs to yogurt or oatmeal.

2.2.17 Turmeric

Nutritional Profile:

Turmeric contains curcumin, known for its anti-inflammatory and antioxidant properties.

Slimming Potential:

Anti-Inflammatory: Curcumin in turmeric may help reduce inflammation, potentially aiding in weight management.

Metabolism Support: Some studies suggest that turmeric may play a role in supporting a healthy metabolism.

Portion/Preparation:

Add turmeric to curries, soups, or make a golden milk latte for a flavorful way to incorporate this spice into your diet.

2.2.18 Goji Berries

Nutritional Profile:

Goji berries are rich in antioxidants, vitamins A and C, fiber, and essential minerals.

Slimming Potential:

Antioxidant Powerhouse: Goji berries' antioxidants may contribute to overall health and well-being.

Fiber Content: Fiber supports digestive health and may aid in weight management.

Portion/Preparation:

Enjoy goji berries as a snack, add them to salads, or include them in trail mixes for a nutrient-packed boost.

2.2.19 Pumpkin Seeds

Nutritional Profile:

Pumpkin seeds are a good source of protein, healthy fats, fiber, and essential minerals.

Slimming Potential:

Protein and Fiber Combo: The protein-fiber combination in pumpkin seeds promotes a feeling of fullness.

Nutrient Density: Pumpkin seeds are nutrient-dense, providing a range of essential minerals.

Portion/Preparation:

A standard serving is around a small handful (about 1 ounce). Sprinkle pumpkin seeds on salads, yogurt, or enjoy them as a standalone snack.

2.2.20 Spirulina

Nutritional Profile:

Spirulina is a blue-green algae rich in protein, vitamins, minerals, and antioxidants.

Slimming Potential:

Protein Power: Spirulina is a complete protein source, supporting muscle maintenance and promoting satiety.

Nutrient Density: Packed with essential nutrients, spirulina offers a concentrated source of nutrition.

Portion/Preparation:

Add spirulina to smoothies, juices, or mix it into yogurt for a nutrient-packed boost.

2.2.21 Acai Berries

Nutritional Profile:

Acai berries are rich in antioxidants, fiber, healthy fats, and essential vitamins.

Slimming Potential:

Antioxidant Rich: Acai berries are known for their high antioxidant content, supporting overall health.

Fiber Boost: The fiber in acai berries aids in digestion and contributes to a feeling of fullness.

Portion/Preparation:

Enjoy acai berries in smoothie bowls, as frozen treats, or add them to your morning yogurt for a delicious and nutritious kick.

2.2.22 Garlic

Nutritional Profile:

Garlic is low in calories and rich in vitamins C and B6, manganese, and antioxidants.

Slimming Potential:

Metabolism Support: Some studies suggest that compounds in garlic may support a healthy metabolism.

Flavorful Substitute: Use garlic to add flavor to dishes without relying on high-calorie sauces or condiments.

Portion/Preparation:

Use garlic in various savory dishes, sauces, or roasted vegetables to benefit from its unique flavor and potential health properties.

2.2.23 Ginger

Nutritional Profile:

Ginger contains bioactive compounds with anti-inflammatory and antioxidant properties.

Slimming Potential:

Digestive Aid: Ginger may help soothe digestive discomfort and reduce inflammation in the gut.

Metabolism Support: Some studies suggest that ginger may contribute to a healthy metabolism.

Portion/Preparation:

Incorporate ginger into teas, stir-fries, or use it as a flavorful spice in both sweet and savory dishes.

2.2.24 Green Tea

Nutritional Profile:

Green tea is rich in antioxidants, particularly catechins, and contains a moderate amount of caffeine.

Slimming Potential:

Catechin Power: The catechins in green tea may support metabolism and contribute to weight management.

Hydration Boost: Choosing green tea over sugary beverages supports hydration without added calories.

Portion/Preparation:

Aim for 2-3 cups of green tea per day. Enjoy it hot or cold, and experiment with different varieties for varied flavors.

2.2.25 Brussels Sprouts

Nutritional Profile:

Brussels sprouts are low in calories and high in fiber, vitamins C and K, and antioxidants.

Slimming Potential:

Fiber Rich: The fiber content in Brussels sprouts promotes a feeling of fullness and supports digestive health.

Nutrient Density: Brussels sprouts provide a range of essential vitamins and minerals.

Portion/Preparation:

Roast, sauté, or steam Brussels sprouts as a delicious side dish, or incorporate them into salads for added crunch and nutrition.

2.2.26 Flaxseeds

Nutritional Profile:

Flaxseeds are rich in omega-3 fatty acids, fiber, and lignans, providing essential nutrients.

Slimming Potential:

Omega-3 Benefits: The omega-3 fatty acids in flaxseeds may support heart health and contribute to a feeling of fullness.

Fiber Boost: The high fiber content aids in digestion and promotes satiety.

Portion/Preparation:

Incorporate flaxseeds into smoothies, sprinkle them on yogurt or oatmeal, or use flaxseed oil in salad dressings.

2.2.27 Mango

Nutritional Profile: Mangoes are rich in vitamins A and C, fiber, and antioxidants.

Slimming Potential:

Fiber Content: The fiber in mangoes promotes a feeling of fullness and supports digestive health.

Natural Sweetness: Mangoes can satisfy sweet cravings in a nutritious way, reducing the need for added sugars.

Portion/Preparation: A serving is typically one cup. Enjoy mangoes as a snack, in smoothies, or as a refreshing addition to salads.

2.2.28 Pomegranate

Nutritional Profile:

Pomegranates are packed with antioxidants, vitamins C and K, and fiber.

Slimming Potential:

Antioxidant Power: Pomegranates' antioxidants may contribute to reducing oxidative stress and supporting overall health.

Fiber Boost: The fiber content aids in digestion and promotes a feeling of fullness.

Portion/Preparation:

Include pomegranate seeds in salads, yogurt, or as a topping for oatmeal for a burst of flavor and nutrition.

2.2.29 Lentils

Nutritional Profile:

Lentils are a rich source of plant-based protein, fiber, and essential vitamins and minerals.

Slimming Potential:

Protein-Fiber Combo: The protein and fiber content in lentils promotes satiety and supports digestive health.

Nutrient Density: Lentils provide a range of essential nutrients with relatively few calories.

Portion/Preparation:

A standard serving is around one cup. Enjoy lentils in soups, stews, salads, or as a side dish for a satisfying meal.

2.2.30 Cabbage

Nutritional Profile:

Cabbage is low in calories and high in fiber, vitamins C and K, and antioxidants.

Slimming Potential:

Low-Calorie Density: Cabbage is a great choice for those looking to manage their weight due to its low-calorie content.

Digestive Health: The fiber in cabbage supports healthy digestion and promotes a feeling of fullness.

Portion/Preparation:

Incorporate cabbage into salads, coleslaw, stir-fries, or soups for a crunchy and nutritious addition to your meals.

2.2.31 Watercress

Nutritional Profile:

Watercress is a leafy green vegetable rich in vitamins A and K, antioxidants, and minerals.

Slimming Potential:

Nutrient Density: Watercress provides a plethora of essential nutrients with minimal calories.

Hydration Boost: As it has a high-water content, it contributes to overall hydration.

Portion/Preparation:

A serving is typically one to two cups. Include watercress in salads, sandwiches, or use it as a garnish for soups.

2.2.32 Cinnamon

Nutritional Profile:

Cinnamon is a spice known for its antioxidant properties and potential health benefits.

Slimming Potential:

Blood Sugar Control: Some studies suggest that cinnamon may help regulate blood sugar levels, aiding in weight management.

Flavorful Substitute: Use cinnamon to add sweetness to dishes without the need for additional sugars.

Portion/Preparation:

Sprinkle cinnamon on oatmeal, yogurt, or use it as a spice in both sweet and savory recipes for added flavor.

2.2.33 Eggs

Nutritional Profile:

Eggs are a complete protein source, containing essential amino acids, healthy fats, and various vitamins.

Slimming Potential:

Protein Powerhouse: The high-quality protein in eggs supports muscle maintenance and promotes a feeling of fullness.

Nutrient-Rich: Eggs provide a range of essential nutrients, including choline, which is important for brain health.

Portion/Preparation:

A serving is typically one to two eggs. Enjoy eggs boiled, poached, scrambled, or as part of omelets for a versatile and nutritious meal.

2.2.34 Tomatoes

Nutritional Profile:

Tomatoes are rich in vitamins A and C, antioxidants, and lycopene.

Slimming Potential:

Low-Calorie: Tomatoes are low in calories, making them a great choice for weight management.

Hydration Support: With high water content, tomatoes contribute to overall hydration.

Portion/Preparation:

Include tomatoes in salads, sauces, soups, or enjoy them fresh as a snack for a burst of flavor and nutrition.

2.2.35 Oranges

Nutritional Profile:

Oranges are a citrus fruit rich in vitamin C, fiber, and antioxidants.

Slimming Potential:

Fiber Boost: The fiber in oranges supports digestive health and promotes a feeling of fullness.

Natural Sweetness: Oranges can satisfy sweet cravings in a nutritious way, reducing the need for added sugars.

Portion/Preparation:

A serving is typically one medium-sized orange. Enjoy oranges as a snack, in fruit salads, or as fresh juice for a refreshing treat.

2.2.36 Arugula

Nutritional Profile:

Arugula is a leafy green vegetable rich in vitamins A, C, and K, as well as antioxidants.

Slimming Potential:

Low-Calorie Density: Arugula is low in calories but high in nutrients, making it an excellent choice for weight management.

Peppery Flavor: The distinct peppery flavor adds a punch to salads and dishes without the need for high-calorie dressings.

Portion/Preparation:

A serving is typically one to two cups. Incorporate arugula into salads, sandwiches, or use it as a pizza or pasta topping.

2.2.37 Brazil Nuts

Nutritional Profile:

Brazil nuts are a rich source of selenium, healthy fats, and essential minerals.

Slimming Potential:

Selenium Content: Selenium may play a role in supporting a healthy metabolism and overall wellness.

Satiety Booster: The combination of healthy fats and protein in Brazil nuts promotes a feeling of fullness.

Portion/Preparation:

A standard serving is around 1-2 nuts. Enjoy Brazil nuts as a snack or include them in mixed nut assortments.

2.2.38 Cranberries

Nutritional Profile:

Cranberries are packed with antioxidants, vitamins C and E, and fiber.

Slimming Potential:

Antioxidant Rich: Cranberries' antioxidants may contribute to reducing oxidative stress, supporting overall health.

Fiber Boost: The fiber content aids in digestion and promotes a feeling of fullness.

Portion/Preparation:

Include cranberries in salads, yogurt, or use them as a topping for oatmeal for a tart and nutritious addition.

2.2.39 Kiwi

Nutritional Profile:

Kiwi is a tropical fruit rich in vitamin C, fiber, and antioxidants.

Slimming Potential:

Fiber Content: The high fiber content in kiwi supports digestive health and promotes a feeling of fullness.

Vitamin C Boost: Kiwi provides a substantial dose of vitamin C, contributing to overall well-being.

Portion/Preparation:

A serving is typically one to two kiwis. Enjoy them fresh as a snack, in fruit salads, or as a colorful addition to desserts.

2.2.40 Hemp Seeds

Nutritional Profile:

Hemp seeds are rich in protein, healthy fats, fiber, and essential minerals.

Slimming Potential:

Protein-Packed: Hemp seeds provide a plant-based protein source, supporting muscle maintenance and satiety.

Omega-3 Fatty Acids: The omega-3s in hemp seeds contribute to heart health and may aid in weight management.

Portion/Preparation:

A standard serving is around 2 tablespoons. Sprinkle hemp seeds on salads, yogurt, or include them in smoothies for an added nutritional boost.

2.2.41 Bell Peppers

Nutritional Profile:

Bell peppers are rich in vitamins A and C, antioxidants, and fiber.

Slimming Potential:

Low-Calorie Density: Bell peppers are low in calories, making them a great choice for weight management.

Colorful Nutrients: The vibrant colors indicate a variety of antioxidants, contributing to overall health.

Portion/Preparation:

A serving is typically one whole pepper. Enjoy bell peppers in salads, stir-fries, or crunchy snacks.

2.2.42 Blackberries

Nutritional Profile:

Blackberries are packed with antioxidants, vitamins C and K, and fiber.

Slimming Potential:

Antioxidant Power: Blackberries' antioxidants may contribute to reducing oxidative stress, supporting overall health.

Fiber Boost: The fiber content aids in digestion and promotes a feeling of fullness.

Portion/Preparation:

A serving is typically one cup. Enjoy blackberries as a snack, in smoothies, or as a topping for yogurt.

2.2.43 Brown Rice

Nutritional Profile:

Brown rice is a whole grain rich in fiber, complex carbohydrates, and various vitamins and minerals.

Slimming Potential:

Sustained Energy: The complex carbs in brown rice provide sustained energy, reducing the likelihood of energy crashes and overeating.

Fiber Content: The fiber content of this food promotes a feeling of fullness and supports digestive health.

Portion/Preparation:

A standard serving is around half to one cup. Use brown rice as a base for stir-fries, bowls, or as a side dish.

2.2.44 Pineapple

Nutritional Profile:

Pineapple is a tropical fruit rich in vitamin C, manganese, and digestive enzymes.

Slimming Potential:

Digestive Enzymes: Bromelain, a digestive enzyme in pineapple, may aid in digestion and reduce bloating.

Natural Sweetness: Pineapple offers a sweet and refreshing flavor without the need for added sugars.

Portion/Preparation: A serving is typically one cup. Enjoy pineapple fresh, in fruit salads, or as a component of refreshing smoothies.

2.2.45 Asparagus

Nutritional Profile: Asparagus is low in calories and high in vitamins A, C, and K, as well as fiber.

Slimming Potential:

Low-Calorie Density: Asparagus is a great choice for those looking to manage their weight due to its low-calorie content.

Nutrient Density: It provides essential nutrients with minimal calories.

Portion/Preparation:

A serving is typically around one cup. Enjoy asparagus grilled, roasted, or steamed as a flavorful and nutritious side dish.

2.2.46 Beetroots

Nutritional Profile:

Beetroots are rich in antioxidants, fiber, vitamins, and minerals.

Slimming Potential:

Antioxidant Power: The antioxidants in beetroots may contribute to reducing oxidative stress and supporting overall health.

Fiber Content: This fruit supports digestive health and helps maintain a feeling of fullness.

Portion/Preparation:

A serving is typically around one cup. Enjoy beetroots roasted, boiled, or grated into salads for a nutritious and colorful addition.

2.2.47 Brussel Sprouts

Nutritional Profile:

Brussels sprouts are low in calories and high in fiber, vitamins C and K, and antioxidants.

Slimming Potential:

Fiber Rich: The fiber content in Brussels sprouts promotes a feeling of fullness and supports digestive health.

Nutrient Density: Brussels sprouts provide a range of essential vitamins and minerals.

Portion/Preparation:

Roast, sauté, or steam Brussels sprouts as a delicious side dish, or incorporate them into salads for added crunch and nutrition.

2.2.48 Chard

Nutritional Profile:

Chard is a leafy green vegetable rich in vitamins A, C, and K, as well as minerals like magnesium and potassium.

Slimming Potential:

Low-Calorie Density: Chard is low in calories but high in nutrients, making it an excellent choice for weight management.

Versatile Greens: Use chard in salads, sautés, or as a nutrient-packed addition to soups and stews.

Portion/Preparation:

A serving is typically one to two cups. Incorporate chard into a variety of dishes for a nutrient boost.

2.2.49 Edamame

Nutritional Profile:

Edamame, or young soybeans, are a rich source of plant-based protein, fiber, and essential vitamins.

Slimming Potential:

Protein-Fiber Combo: The protein and fiber content in edamame promotes satiety and supports digestive health.

Nutrient-Rich Snack: Enjoy edamame as a wholesome and satisfying snack.

Portion/Preparation:

A standard serving is around one cup. Boil or steam edamame and sprinkle with a pinch of salt for a nutritious snack.

2.2.50 Raspberries

Nutritional Profile:

Raspberries are rich in antioxidants, fiber, vitamins C and K, and essential minerals.

Slimming Potential:

Antioxidant Power: Raspberries' antioxidants may contribute to reducing oxidative stress, supporting overall health.

Fiber Boost: The fiber content aids in digestion and promotes a feeling of fullness.

Portion/Preparation:

A serving is typically one cup. Enjoy raspberries as a snack, in smoothies, or as a topping for yogurt.

2.3 Interconnection of the Superfoods: A Quantum Synergy

Beyond their individual merits, Quantum Slimming Superfoods share a unique synergy when combined. The interconnection of Quantum Slimming Superfoods lies in their collective ability to contribute to a holistic and sustainable approach to weight loss. These superfoods, carefully curated for their nutritional richness, share common characteristics that make them unique and effective in supporting weight management. Here's why they stand out:

1. Nutrient Density:

Common Trait: All these superfoods are nutrient-dense, meaning they pack a significant number of vitamins, minerals, and antioxidants relative to their calorie content.

Unique Impact: This nutrient density ensures that your body receives essential nutrients even in a calorie-controlled diet, preventing nutrient deficiencies often associated with restrictive eating.

2. High Fiber Content:

Common Trait: Most of these superfoods are rich in dietary fiber.

Unique Impact: Fiber promotes a feeling of fullness, reduces overall calorie intake, and supports digestive health. This satiety effect is crucial for weight loss as it helps control portion sizes and minimizes overeating.

3. Protein-Rich Selection:

Common Trait: Several superfoods, such as nuts, seeds, and legumes, provide a notable amount of protein.

Unique Impact: Protein is essential for muscle maintenance and repair. Including protein-rich foods in your diet helps preserve lean muscle mass during weight loss, ensuring that the body primarily sheds fat.

4. Omega-3 Fatty Acids:

Common Trait: Certain superfoods like chia seeds, flaxseeds, and fatty fish (salmon) are rich in omega-3 fatty acids.

Unique Impact: Omega-3s play a role in reducing inflammation, supporting metabolic health, and contributing to a sense of fullness, which are all beneficial for weight loss.

5. Low-Calorie Density:

Common Trait: Many of these superfoods, including leafy greens, berries, and cruciferous vegetables, are low in calories.

Unique Impact: Foods with low-calorie density allow for larger portions without excessive calorie intake. This aids in managing hunger while still adhering to a calorie-controlled diet.

6. Antioxidant-Rich Profile:

Common Trait: Berries, dark leafy greens, and colorful vegetables are packed with antioxidants.

Unique Impact: Antioxidants combat oxidative stress, promoting overall health. This is particularly relevant during weight loss, as the body undergoes metabolic changes that can generate free radicals.

7. Balanced Macronutrients:

Common Trait: These superfoods collectively provide a balanced mix of carbohydrates, proteins, and healthy fats.

Unique Impact: A balanced macronutrient profile ensures sustained energy levels, preventing energy crashes and the subsequent impulse to consume high-calorie snacks.

8. Natural Sweetness:

Common Trait: Fruits like berries, mangoes, and oranges contribute natural sweetness.

Unique Impact: The natural sugars in these fruits offer a sweet taste without the added sugars found in many processed foods, making them a healthier choice for those with a sweet tooth.

9. Metabolism Support:

Common Trait: Some superfoods, like green tea, turmeric, and certain nuts, have compounds believed to support metabolism.

Unique Impact: These foods may contribute to enhanced calorie burning, making weight loss more efficient.

Chapter Three
The Quantum Slimming Lifestyle

In the pursuit of the Quantum Slimming lifestyle, this chapter serves as a comprehensive guide, encompassing the seamless integration of superfoods into your daily diet, exploring the synergies between Quantum Slimming Superfoods, and providing invaluable lifestyle tips for enhancing weight loss results.

A. Incorporating Superfoods into Your Daily Diet

3.1 Embracing Nutrient-Rich Habits

Explore the diverse array of Quantum Slimming Superfoods and discover inventive ways to incorporate them into your daily meals. From vibrant salads featuring leafy greens to nutrient-packed smoothies blending berries and chia seeds, the possibilities are as diverse as the superfoods themselves. This section provides practical insights and culinary inspiration to make these nutritional powerhouses a delightful part of your everyday diet.

3.2 Culinary Creativity with Quantum Slimming Superfoods

Unlock the full potential of Quantum Slimming Superfoods by experimenting with innovative recipes. Dive into the art of combining flavors, textures, and colors to create meals that not only support your weight loss goals but also tantalize your taste buds. From savory dishes featuring salmon and asparagus to sweet treats with mango and yogurt, this section encourages culinary creativity while adhering to the principles of Quantum Slimming.

B. Synergies Between Quantum Slimming Superfoods

3.3 The Art of Complementary Pairing

Explore the intricate synergies between Quantum Slimming Superfoods, understanding how their combined forces can amplify their individual benefits. Learn about pairing complementary superfoods to enhance nutrient absorption and create a harmonious balance of flavors. Uncover the science behind these synergies and how they contribute to the overarching goal of effective weight management.

3.4 Crafting Balanced Meals with Superfood Harmony

Delve into the principles of meal balance, incorporating various superfoods to create nutritionally complete and satisfying dishes. Understand how proteins, carbohydrates, and healthy fats from different superfoods can work in tandem to support energy levels, satiety, and overall well-being.

This section provides practical tips for structuring meals that harness the synergistic powers of Quantum Slimming Superfoods.

C. Lifestyle Tips for Enhancing Weight Loss Results

3.5 Mindful Living Practices

Explore the profound impact of mindfulness on your Quantum Slimming journey. Learn techniques for cultivating mindfulness in your daily life, from mindful eating practices to incorporating mindful movement. Understand how these practices not only enhance the weight loss experience but also contribute to a holistic sense of well-being.

3.6 Physical Activity and Quantum Slimming

Uncover the symbiotic relationship between physical activity and Quantum Slimming. Discover the types of exercises that complement your weight loss goals and how consistent movement contributes to overall health. This section provides practical suggestions for incorporating enjoyable physical activities into your routine, creating a balanced and sustainable approach to fitness.

3.7 Optimizing Sleep for Quantum Slimming

Recognize the pivotal role of sleep in the Quantum Slimming lifestyle. Understand how quality sleep supports hormonal balance, metabolism, and the body's natural processes for weight management. Gain insights into optimizing your sleep environment and developing healthy sleep habits to maximize the effectiveness of your Quantum Slimming journey. Additionally, discover the profound connection between well-rested nights and improved decision-making, stress resilience, and overall mental well-being, underscoring the integral role of sleep in achieving holistic health and weight loss success.

Chapter Four
Quantum Slimming: Success Stories

Let us embark on a journey through tangible victories and heartfelt testimonials where Quantum Slimming transcends theory to become a transformative force in the lives of individuals who embraced superfoods and navigated seamless weight loss journeys.

A. Real-Life Experiences with Quantum Slimming

4.1 Unveiling the Real Transformations

Meet Sarah, a busy professional who, by incorporating Quantum Slimming Superfoods into her daily meals, witnessed a remarkable transformation. Balancing a hectic schedule, she embraced nutrient-rich foods like kale, berries, and lean proteins. Through mindful eating and a commitment to her Quantum Slimming Meal Plan, Sarah not only shed excess weight but also experienced heightened energy levels and mental clarity.

4.2 John's Journey to Health

Discover John's journey, where the integration of Quantum Slimming Superfoods became a game-changer. John, a father of two, found solace in the simplicity of whole foods. By savoring delicious recipes featuring a mix of superfoods like salmon, quinoa, and vibrant vegetables, he achieved sustainable weight loss. John's story highlights the practicality of Quantum Slimming amid a bustling family life.

B. Testimonials from Individuals Who Defied Gravity in Their Weight Loss Journey

4.3 A Testimony of Transformation

Read Emily's testimony—a poignant narrative of resilience and transformation. Through embracing the Quantum Slimming lifestyle, Emily discovered a renewed sense of self. Her testimonial speaks of the emotional and mental well-being that accompanied her physical transformation. Emily's journey exemplifies the holistic impact of Quantum Slimming on one's overall quality of life.

4.4 Celebrating Everyday Triumphs

Join Mark on his Quantum Slimming odyssey—a celebration of everyday triumphs. By incorporating superfoods into his routine, Mark not only achieved weight loss but also found joy in adopting a healthier lifestyle. His testimonial reflects the ripple effect of positive changes, from improved sleep to enhanced mood, showcasing the domino of benefits that follow a Quantum Slimming journey.

Chapter Five
Overcoming Challenges

Navigating the quantum slimming journey involves acknowledging and surmounting obstacles that commonly accompany weight loss. This section delves into addressing common weight loss obstacles and offers practical tips and strategies to fortify your commitment to the Quantum Slimming lifestyle.

Addressing Common Weight Loss Obstacles

5.1 The Plateau Predicament

Encountering plateaus is a shared experience on the weight loss path. We unravel the science behind plateaus and provide insights into adjusting your quantum slimming approach to overcome these temporary halts. Discover strategies to reignite progress and sustain your momentum.

5.2 Social Challenges and Celebrations

Navigating social situations and celebratory events while adhering to a Quantum Slimming lifestyle can be challenging. Learn how to gracefully navigate gatherings, make mindful choices, and maintain your commitment to healthier living without feeling deprived.

5.3 Emotional Eating and Stress

Emotional eating often poses a significant hurdle. We explore the link between emotions and eating habits, providing practical tools to identify triggers and develop healthier coping mechanisms. Address stressors proactively to cultivate a resilient mindset on your weight loss journey.

Tips and Strategies for Staying Committed to the Quantum Slimming Lifestyle

5.4 Mindful Meal Planning

Crafting a mindful meal plan is essential for long-term success. Uncover strategies for effective meal planning, grocery shopping, and preparation, ensuring that Quantum Slimming seamlessly integrates into your lifestyle without becoming a source of stress.

5.5 Consistency in Quantum Superfood Selection

Maintaining consistency in selecting Quantum Slimming Superfoods is key. We provide guidance on diversifying your superfood choices, preventing monotony, and optimizing nutritional intake for sustained energy and vitality.

5.6 Building a Support System

Forge connections with like-minded individuals embarking on their quantum slimming journey. Building a support system fosters accountability, encouragement, and shared experiences. Learn how to leverage community support to enhance your commitment and resilience.

5.7 The Role of Mindfulness in Quantum Slimming

Explore the transformative impact of mindfulness on staying committed to quantum slimming. Discover mindfulness practices that extend beyond mealtime, contributing to a balanced and harmonious lifestyle. Cultivate an awareness that aligns with your weight loss goals.

Chapter Six
Beyond the Scale

In this concluding chapter, we transcend the numerical focus of weight loss and delve into the holistic health benefits of quantum slimming. Beyond the scale, we explore the profound impact that the Quantum Slimming lifestyle, enriched by superfood nutrition, has on enhancing overall well-being.

Exploring the Holistic Health Benefits of Quantum Slimming

6.1 Vibrant Energy and Vitality

Experience a surge in vibrant energy and vitality as you embrace the Quantum Slimming journey. The nutrient-dense superfoods incorporated into your daily meals contribute essential vitamins and minerals, promoting sustained energy levels throughout the day. Say goodbye to energy slumps and welcome a renewed sense of vigor.

6.2 Mental Clarity and Focus

Discover the cognitive benefits of quantum slimming as superfoods nourish not just your body but also your mind.

Essential fatty acids, antioxidants, and a balanced intake of nutrients support mental clarity and focus. Experience improved concentration and cognitive function, unlocking your full potential in daily tasks and challenges.

6.3 Radiant Skin and Hair

Uncover the beauty-enhancing effects of Quantum Slimming Superfoods. Packed with antioxidants, these superfoods combat oxidative stress, promoting healthy skin and a radiant complexion. Notice improvements in hair health, as the nourishing elements contribute to strength and luster from within.

Enhancing Overall Well-Being Through Superfood Nutrition

6.4 Gut Health and Digestive Harmony

A harmonious digestive system is paramount for overall well-being. Quantum Slimming Superfoods, rich in fiber and probiotics, foster a healthy gut environment. Experience improved digestion, reduced bloating, and enhanced nutrient absorption, laying the foundation for optimal health.

6.5 Immune System Resilience

Elevate your immune system's resilience with the immune-boosting properties of Quantum Slimming Superfoods. The diverse array of vitamins, minerals, and antioxidants fortify your body's defense mechanisms, supporting your ability to ward off illnesses and infections.

6.6 Emotional Well-Being and Mood Stability

Nourish not only your body but also your emotional well-being through quantum slimming. Superfoods contribute to mood stability by providing essential nutrients that support neurotransmitter function. Experience a positive impact on your overall emotional balance and well-being.

6.7 Sustainable, Healthy Lifestyle Habits

Embrace the sustainability of quantum slimming as a lifestyle. Beyond weight loss, these habits foster long-term well-being. Discover the joy of mindful eating, the empowerment of regular physical activity, and the importance of quality sleep as integral components of a holistic and sustainable lifestyle.

Conclusion

Summing Up the Quantum Slimming Journey

As we draw the curtains on the Quantum Slimming journey, it's time to reflect on the transformative odyssey you've embarked upon. Throughout this comprehensive guide, you've delved into the world of quantum slimming, embracing nutrient-dense superfoods, and fostering a holistic approach to well-being. From the initial exploration of potent superfoods to the practical implementation of a Quantum Slimming Meal Plan, your journey has been one of discovery, resilience, and positive change.

Encouragement and Inspiration for Readers

To every reader who has ventured through these pages, your commitment to exploring a healthier lifestyle is commendable. Take a moment to acknowledge the strides you've made, both big and small. The Quantum Slimming journey is not just about shedding pounds; it's about cultivating sustainable habits, nurturing overall well-being, and unlocking the full potential of your vitality. Remember, each step forward is a victory, and your journey is uniquely yours.

Looking Ahead: The Future of Quantum Slimming

As we look ahead, envision the future of your Quantum Slimming lifestyle. The principles you've embraced—mindful eating, superfood nutrition, and holistic well-being—are not just temporary measures but enduring pillars of a vibrant life. Continue to explore new superfoods, experiment with recipes, and stay attuned to the needs of your body. The journey doesn't end here; it evolves with you, adapting to the seasons of your life.

In the pages of this guide, you've discovered the potential for positive change within yourself. Carry the lessons, the recipes, and the inspiration with you as you navigate the chapters of your life. Whether you're maintaining your achieved goals or pushing new boundaries, the Quantum Slimming philosophy remains a guiding light for a flourishing and balanced existence.

As you step forward from this conclusion, may you continue to thrive, embodying the essence of quantum slimming—where health, energy, and well-being converge into a symphony of vitality. The future is yours to shape, and with the principles of quantum slimming as your guide, it promises to be a journey filled with strength, resilience, and a profound connection to your own flourishing health.

Appendix

Weekly Quantum Slimming Meal Plan

Sunday		Water Intake	Exercise	Notes
B	Quantum Superfood Sunday: Whole-grain pancakes made with mashed banana and walnuts. Drizzled with maple syrup.	♡		
L	Quantum Superfood Salad: Kale and mixed greens topped with strawberries, blueberries, walnuts, and a lemon-poppy seed dressing.	♡		
D	Quantum Baked Cod with Turmeric: Baked cod fillet seasoned with turmeric and served with quinoa and roasted Brussels sprouts.	♡		
Monday		♡		
B	Quantum Greens Galore: Oats cooked with green tea, topped with sliced kiwi, almonds, and a drizzle of honey.	♡		
L	Quantum Chickpea and Spinach Curry: Chickpeas and spinach	♡		

	cooked in a flavorful curry sauce, served with brown rice.			
D	Vegetable Stir-Fry: Colorful vegetable stir-fry with tofu, sesame seeds, and a soy-ginger sauce. Served over quinoa	♡		
Tuesday		♡		
B	Quantum Power Breakfast: Whole-grain toast topped with mashed avocado, a poached egg, cherry tomatoes, and a sprinkle of black pepper.	♡		
L	Quantum Lentil Soup: Hearty lentil soup with carrots, celery, tomatoes, and kale. Accompanied by a side of whole-grain bread.	♡		
D	Quantum Grilled Chicken Salad Grilled chicken breast over a bed of mixed greens, cherry tomatoes, bell peppers, and a balsamic vinaigrette.	♡		
Wednesday		♡		
B	Quantum Fusion Feast: Chia seeds soaked in almond milk and layered with mango chunks. Garnished with a dollop of Greek yogurt.	♡		

L	Quantum Quinoa Bowl: Quinoa bowl with black beans, corn, avocado, cherry tomatoes, and cilantro. Drizzled with lime dressing.	♡		
D	Quantum Sweet Potato and Kale Stir-Fry: Stir-fried sweet potatoes, kale, and tofu in a sesame-ginger sauce. Served over brown rice.	♡		
Thursday		♡		
B	Quantum Delightful Dishes: Acai bowl topped with banana slices, almond butter, granola, and a sprinkle of coconut flakes.	♡		
L	Quantum Mediterranean Wrap: Whole-grain wrap filled with hummus, falafel, cucumber, tomatoes, and shredded lettuce.	♡		
D	Quantum Roasted Veggie Pizza: Whole-grain pizza crust topped with tomato sauce, roasted vegetables, feta cheese, and a drizzle of olive oil.	♡		
Friday		♡		

B	Quantum Energizing Eats: Greek yogurt layered with mixed berries, granola, and a dollop of honey.	♡		
L	Quantum Spinach and Feta Stuffed Chicken Breast: Chicken breast stuffed with spinach and feta, served with quinoa and steamed green beans.	♡		
D	Quantum Shrimp and Broccoli Stir-Fry: Shrimp and broccoli stir-fried in a garlic-ginger sauce, served over brown rice.	♡		
Saturday	♡			
B	Quantum Berry Smoothie Bowl: Blend mixed berries, spinach, chia seeds, and almond milk. Top with sliced banana, granola, and a sprinkle of pumpkin seeds.	♡		
L	Quantum Quinoa Salad: Quinoa mixed with cherry tomatoes, cucumber, avocado, feta cheese, and a lemon-tahini dressing.	♡		
D	Quantum Baked Salmon:	♡		

	Baked salmon fillet seasoned with turmeric and served with roasted sweet potatoes and steamed broccoli.			

Instructions:
Exercise: Record any physical activity or exercise you engage in each day.
Water Intake: Track your daily water consumption.
Notes: Use this section to jot down any observations, challenges, or positive experiences during the day.

www.ingramcontent.com/pod-product-compliance
Lightning Source LLC
Chambersburg PA
CBHW071059260726
48661CB00006B/2357